MY CHARCOT FOOT STORY

By John P. Creed

PREFACE

This book represents a timeline and a recollection of events beginning in 2016 that ultimately led to the below the knee amputation of my left leg in 2020. My goal is to educate and inform people of the symptoms, causes and treatment of Charcot Foot or Charcot Arthropathy.

WARNING

This book will contain graphic pictures of my actual injuries and x-rays displaying open wounds, blood, stitches and surgical repairs throughout my ordeal. I will tell the story, to the best of my recollection, with explanations and definitions as they were told to me by my Medical Teams with some referencing and I will throw a bit of humor in as well.

CHAPTERS

1. Who am I?
2. What is Charcot Arthropathy (Charcot Foot)?
3. 2016-2017 For Whom the Bell "Toes"
4. 2018-2019 Free Fallin'
5. 2020 Bye, Bye Leg
6. 2021 to present
7. Thank you

Chapter 1: Who am I?

A little bit about myself. I was born in the town of Plymouth, Massachusetts. I lived and grew up on the South Shore area of Boston in Green Harbor, which is a section of Marshfield. I am one of eight siblings. My father was a man who believed that whatever type of home repair it was, he could fix it. I guess that's the upside to having eight kids. He had his own work force.

From an early age my older brothers would handle the larger projects my father planned out such as shingling a new roof, digging a new leeching field for the septic system and digging through the basement concrete to install a French drain. My younger brother, Eddie, and me were responsible for all landscaping, mowing, linseed oiling the wooden gutters and a bit of painting.

My family was well known in the community and my father would often send me and my brother to the homes of the elderly and the church nun to rake leaves, shovel snow and mow lawns. When we were twelve, we had quite a substantial little mowing service. One summer when the town was installing a public septic system, each home was responsible for getting their own septic lines connected to the town service. We had three pine trees well over sixty feet high on the side of our house and one of them was in direct line with the hookup location. My father wanted to save the roots of the tree, so we had to dig under the massive root system of the pine tree in the middle of the summer. The ditch started at a four-foot depth along the foundation down to eleven feet at the connection site. Unfortunately, a couple of years later, my father decided to cut the trees down because they were getting too big, but it was just our luck that the project took place when it did. What a blast we had when, after the trees were removed, my father had us go over to the neighbor's farm after school with five-gallon buckets to cut out and transplant grass to create a lawn that the trees had destroyed over the years. Yippee!

The point I'm trying to make is that I am no stranger to hard work. I carry those fundamentals to this day and that's what ultimately led me to establishing my own business after years of working with one of my brothers in the painting and home improvements field. At one point I moved to Pennsylvania and established my own company of painting and home repairs. I worked on many projects such as painting, tiling, power washing, kitchen and bath remodels, construction with some electrical and plumbing work as well. I tried not to leave much to chance and believed there was not much I could not handle by myself. Hard work is medicine for the soul but sometimes that hard work would lead to injuries and wear and tear on the body over time. As you will read in the upcoming chapters, that hard work and wear and tear eventually caught up to me.

In 1993 I was diagnosed with Type II Diabetes after becoming very sick and losing 120lbs. I went to a Diabetic Teaching Hospital to learn about this illness and how to control it. For the next 10 years I managed my condition with diet and exercise and took no medication. It was the healthiest time of my adult life. As you read on you will see that things changed over time

Chapter 2: What is Charcot Arthropathy (Charcot Foot)?

Over the past several years when I have explained to some healthcare professionals that I have (or had) Charcot foot they would look at me as if either a) they have never heard of it or b) they have heard of it but don't necessarily understand the scope of the condition. Now, to be clear, Charcot Foot is **not** to be confused with Charcot Marie Tooth disease. If you "Google" the word Charcot, mostly Charcot Marie Tooth sites are called up. They share some similar symptoms, but they have their own identities.

Charcot-Marie-Tooth disease is a group of disorders that cause nerve damage. This damage is mostly in the arms and legs (peripheral nerves). Charcot-Marie-Tooth disease is also called hereditary motor and sensory neuropathy.

Charcot-Marie-Tooth disease results in smaller, weaker muscles. You may also experience loss of sensation and muscle contractions, and difficulty walking. Foot deformities are common. Symptoms usually begin in the feet and legs, but they may eventually affect your hands and arms.

Symptoms of Charcot-Marie-Tooth disease typically appear in early adulthood but may also develop later in life. People may experience high foot arches, hammertoes, clumsiness or constant tripping, loss of muscle in the legs and feet, weakness in lower extremities or even curvature of the spine. Those afflicted may also experience a loss of ability to run or exercise, dropfoot and increased weakness and general fatigue. As Charcot-Marie-Tooth disease progresses, symptoms may spread from the feet and legs to the upper extremities. Charcot-Marie-Tooth disease is a genetic condition that occurs when there are mutations in the genes that affect the nerves in your feet, legs, hands and arms. It is hereditary so you may be prone to the disease if anyone in your immediate family has it. It is a rare condition that less than 200,000 people per year are diagnosed with most subjects having neuropathy and or diabetes.

What Is Charcot Foot?

Charcot foot is a condition causing weakening of the bones in the foot that can occur in people who have significant nerve damage. Bones become weakened enough to fracture, and splinter simply by continued walking, which can lead to deformities. As it progresses, the joints collapse and the foot takes on an abnormal shape, creating a rocker-bottom foot deformity.

Charcot foot is a serious condition that can lead to severe deformity, disability and even amputation. Because of its seriousness, it is important that patients living with diabetes or neuropathy take preventive measures and seek immediate care if signs or symptoms appear.

Charcot foot develops as a result of neuropathy, which decreases sensation to the feet. It is common for people to walk on a fractured or broken foot without feeling a thing, which makes the situation worse. When I had my surgery, the doctor asked me if I had broken my foot before. I told him no, but he said that all of my metatarsals were curved as if they broke and healed with this curvature. People with peripheral neuropathy are at risk for developing Charcot foot, especially over time and lack of proper care. When it is present your feet would feel warm to the touch, soreness, redness and swelling and increased pain. Checking your feet often for unexplained bruising or blisters or any unusual signs is important in early diagnosis.

Early diagnosis of Charcot foot is extremely important for successful treatment. To determine a diagnosis the doctor will ask about your history with the foot or ankle such as past injuries or fractures. It is common to order x-rays and imaging of both feet and ankles for inspection and comparison images to review for aspect changes.

It is extremely important to follow a doctors treatment plan for Charcot foot. Failure to do so can lead to the loss of a toe, foot, leg or life. Treatment for Charcot foot is relative to a patient's severity of symptoms or stage of the affliction. In my case, my doctor prescribed special orthotic inserts and shoes. These items assisted in the support and comfort of my foot. Some people may be told to stay off their feet for an indefinite period until bones that are broken or fractured can heal or the condition pauses. Some need complete immobilization of the leg or foot with the use of leg braces and casting to protect from further damage. Bones can heal themselves but how long that can take varies from person to person. When Charcot is diagnosed early you would be told to limit activities especially if you are very active and exercise frequently. Staying off your feet could be key to limiting pain and the worsening of the condition.

Preventative measures for people at risk of Charcot foot include maintaining a healthy lifestyle and low glucose blood levels. Daily foot inspections. Maintaining a healthy weight and no extreme exercise or outdoor activities. Exercise is good but nothing too extreme. If you are a diabetic or have neuropathy it is important to have either a podiatrist or foot and ankle specialist that you see to be monitored for changes or symptoms. Both types of Physicians are well trained in foot and ankle issues. The surgeon specialist will be more qualified for issues related to Charcot deformities and persons who are already in the early stages of the illness and could assist in maintenance of the condition. The Podiatrist would be a good option if you are at high risk for Charcot and would assist in managing a planned and healthy regimen for prevention and care.

Now that the explanations, definitions and most related information for both conditions have been presented I will tell you of my own personal history that led to my diagnosis and how and why I made the decisions I made.

Chapter 3: 2016 -2017 For Whom the Bell "Toes"

If pain, bad luck and bad timing were a lottery prize I'd be a millionaire. The order in which these events occurred will tell a tale that shaped my future and will help you understand my thought process in making decisions.

In the fall of 2016, I was a busy contractor with a full schedule. At the time, I had a two-man crew of experienced Painters that assisted me in completing multiple jobs. I was a "Jack of all trades" kind of guy as I had a lot of experience in carpentry and home improvements along with my skills as a Professional Painter. My crew did not have the carpentry skills that I possessed so when a painting project included any home repairs or carpentry issues, I would tackle those projects by myself and would let the guys focus on the painting.

I had recently moved into a new apartment and was putting furniture in place for my bedroom, living room and office. Some of the bookcases and shelving units came with very small screws to use in the construction of the furniture. Now I am a firm believer on getting the proper footwear for work vs play with comfort being a priority. The footwear I had on the day I put the furniture together had a memory type insole that was very comfortable. Being a Type II Diabetic has its related problems. One such problem is peripheral neuropathy which meant that over time I experienced nerve damage which caused pain and numbness in my hands and feet. One example of loss of sensation in my feet was when I stepped on a large 10d nail. What alerted me to this was that when I took a step, the 2x4 the nail was attached to was also attached to my foot through the sole of the shoe. When I took a step, the board was nailed into my foot, and I did not know it until I started walking and the board went with me. I did not feel it at all.

About a month after I put the furniture together, I noticed at the end of the workday that I had a small amount of blood on my left sock where the big toe was. I thought nothing of it as I had very dry and cracked feet from the work I was doing. But every day the blood spots were more frequent. Being a diabetic, I conducted foot inspections occasionally because of the neuropathy as directed by podiatrists over the years. My big toe always looked ugly because of the "carpenters' foot" syndrome I was so thrilled to have (that's sarcasm). So, the feet always looked dry, cracked and nasty. One day, when I was on a job, my toe was bothering me a bit so I decided to remove my shoe and have a look. This is what I saw.

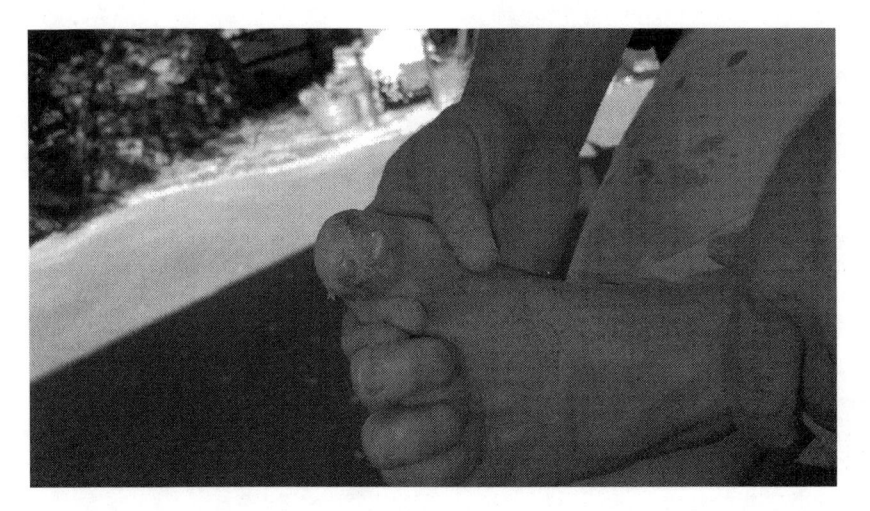

Notice the Inflammation and rough skin. Because of the constant blood spot on my sock, I thought that maybe I stepped on a nail or perhaps something inside the shoe was irritating my toe. When I did an inspection of the shoe, I was shocked to find a small furniture screw, from my apartment, was lodged in the memory foam sole of my shoe where the big toe was located. I freaked out a bit and decided to get an emergency appointment with my podiatrist. Now people "peel" many things in life. People can peel a banana, apple skin or an orange to name a few. But a toe? Yup. A toe. When my podiatrist completed his inspection, he told me that I had a hole, about the size of a dime, that was underneath the hard skin layer of my big toe and that the blood was seeping out from underneath. And so, for the wound to heal properly he had to take steps to ensure that outcome. He had to……wait for it……. can you guess? Exactly. He had to "peel" that rough layer of nasty skin off to reveal the wound and then treat the spot in order to promote the healing process and new healthy skin. Right then and there, in his office, he took out a scalpel and proceeded to cut around the circumference of my toe and peel off the bad layer of skin. Cringe moment number one. I was advised to stay off my feet for a bit to allow the wound to heal. I stayed off my foot for a month. The hole in my toe got smaller. The picture shown is the best that t̶̶̶̶̶̶̶̶̶̶̶̶̶̶̶̶̶̶̶̶̶̶̶̶̶̶̶̶̶̶k.

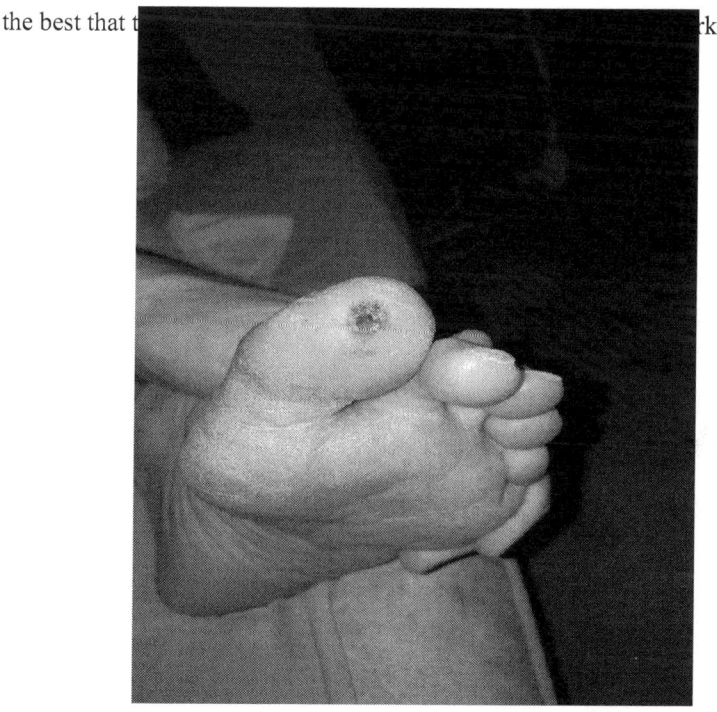

#/ preface / 10

Unfortunately, "when the cat's away the mice will play". My jobs were slowing down. The guys were hard workers but when I was not on the job the work took longer to complete and I was struggling to pay bills. I had to go back to work. The next series of pictures will show how   r a ten-month period.

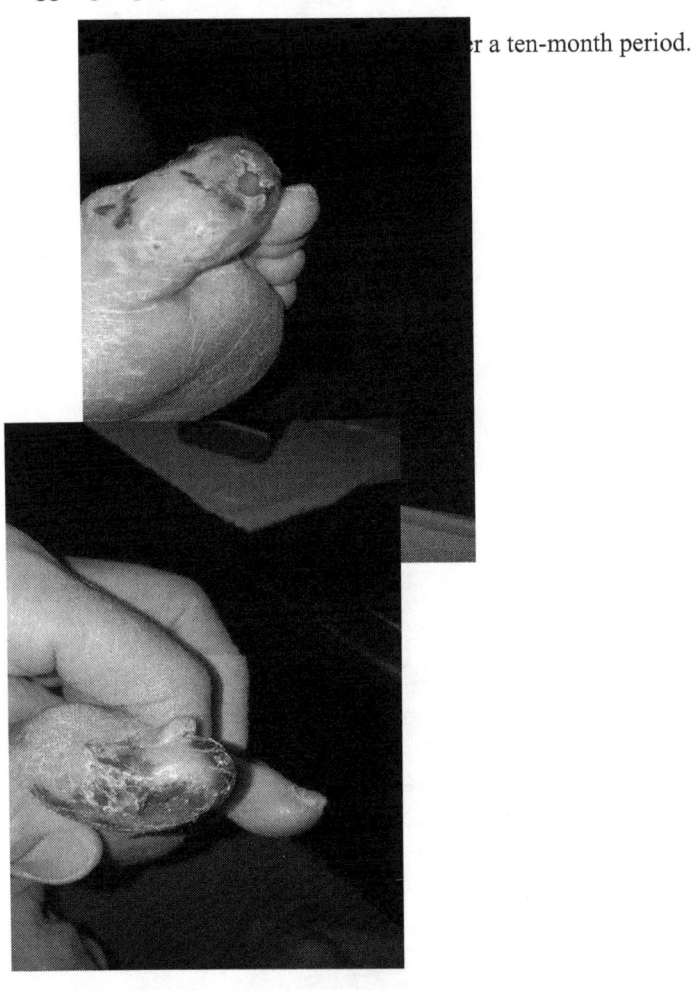

/ preface / 11

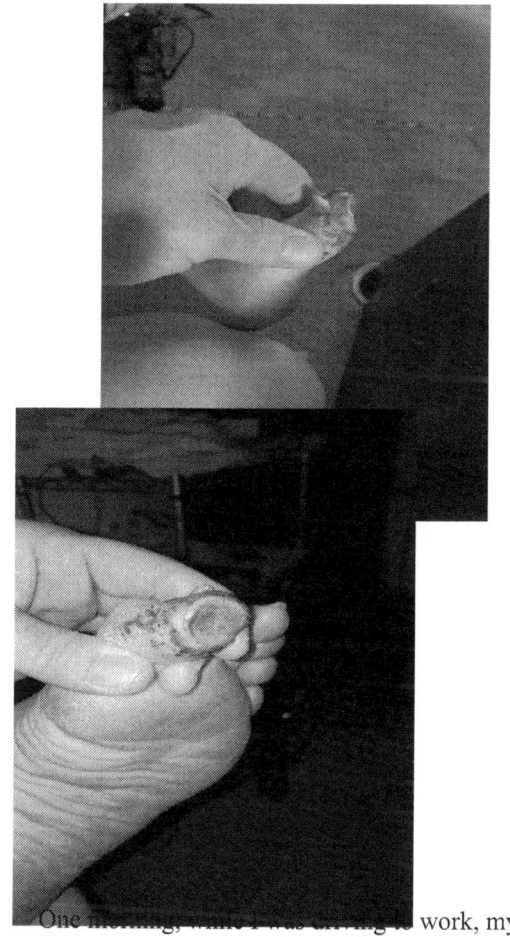

One morning, while I was driving to work, my left leg started to swell. The swelling went all the way up to my groin area. I drove myself to the E.R. The staff at the hospital did x-rays and used an ultrasound machine on the lymph nodes around my groin. The diagnosis was osteomyelitis in my left toe. The infection in my toe had gotten into the bone. I had 2 choices. Insert a "pig tail" in my elbow for infusions of I.V. antibiotics for weeks to combat the infection. The other option was to remove the toe. The concerns were that the antibiotics were not a guarantee that it would eliminate the infection and that the osteomyelitis could progress further in the bones and could lead to removal of my leg. For me, the choice was obvious.

/ preface / 12

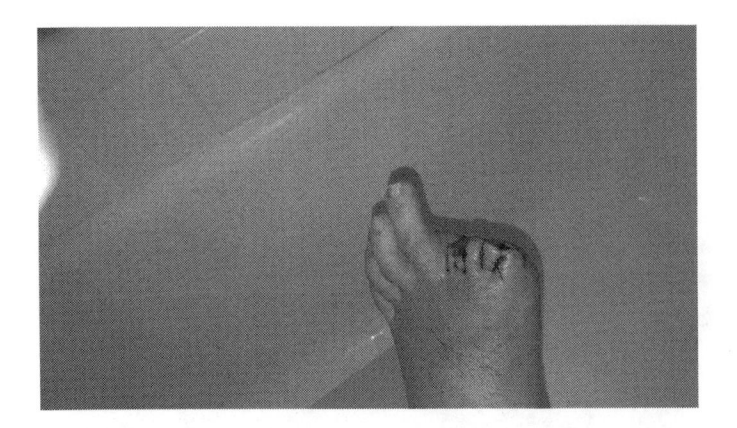

Cringe moment number two. The foot healed in a few weeks, and I was back on the job. People have no idea how important your big toe is. It handles the weight of your body when walking and provides overall balance and stability. Without it you will end up with the next issue.

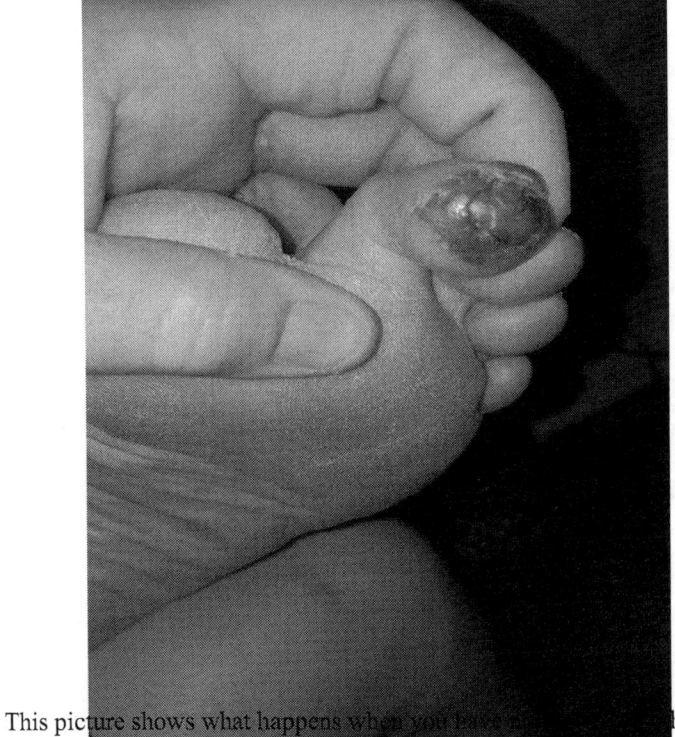

This picture shows what happens when you have no toe. The next in line smaller toe must handle the weight and balance of your body. I came close to losing that toe. The solution was an orthotic insert for my shoes that had a "false toe" installed in the void area of the insert where my big toe would have been. I was amazed at how important your big toe is based on how many times I almost fell flat on my face or tripped or scuffed my shoe. After my podiatrist "snipped" the tendon in that toe to straighten it out, the orthotics worked like magic in the healing that issue.

Chapter 4; 2018-2019 Free Fallin'

In the fall of 2018, I was on an extension ladder approximately 8-10 feet high from the bottom of the driveway. Now I have been climbing ladders for 30 years. I've been higher than 40 feet on many occasions. I've been in scary ladder situations that would make a novice painter quit if they had to climb to such heights (it's happened a couple of times). So, when I went up that ladder it was no big deal as I had done it thousands of times. To this day I still can't say why or what caused the ladder to move. When placing an extension ladder against a sidewall of a home, you would face the ladder towards the wall, move it back to an appropriate distance for a proper angle as you slowly move the top of the ladder to softly land on the wall. The top rails of the ladder had rubber ladder "mitts" on them so as not to scratch or damage the sidewall and prevent the top of the ladder from sliding. Next you would adjust the bottom "feet" of the ladder appropriately, so the angle was not too steep. The feet of the ladder have a rubber strip on the bottom to prevent slippage or movement while working. The feet can also be turned back to rest on the bottom rail which allows for the "claw" like toes of the feet to be dug into dirt to lock the ladder into the ground and adjust when leveling the bottom.

When I started climbing the ladder, always maintaining 3 points of contact, I got about 8 feet in the air when the unthinkable happened. The bottom of the ladder "kicked out" backwards which made the top of the ladder slide down the face of the sidewall. I had my hands on the top rails, my feet on a rung, or step of the ladder, and my knees resting on the rung above as I" rode" the ladder to the pavement. The impact was violent. Imagine the force of my 235-pound weight and the angle of the ladder as it slammed on the ground. The impact literally bounced me in the air, and I landed next to the ladder. At that point I thought I had either broken my leg or my knee cap. My whole body was in pain. I rolled over to a sitting position and just sat there and assessed the situation. I knew I was injured but I did not know the extent of the damage. I knew my leg had issues so when I got my composure back, I noticed my left knee was not where I had last left it. Instead of being in its usual location it was now on the side of my leg. Hmm, that's not right. My hands and wrists hurt, my back hurt, my arms and shoulders hurt, and my feet were throbbing. I tried to stand up, but my left leg was not moving and any attempt to do so was met by the most extreme pain I had ever felt in my life. The leg was deadweight at this point. I scooted on my but to the tailgate of my truck, which was behind me, and grabbed on and lifted myself up with my right leg, which hurt like hell, but at least I could stand on it. I sat on the tailgate and gathered myself again. I could not walk on my left leg, so I tried to hop to get to the cab of the truck and again, excruciating pain. I reached down with my left hand, grabbed ahold of my shoelaces and lifted my left leg, hopped on my right foot while leaning on the truck and somehow got myself into the cab of the truck and drove myself to the Emergency room. Not a pleasant ride I can tell you.

The Emergency room at the hospital I drove to, had a valet service. I pulled up and told the guys on duty that I had a bad fall and could not walk. They brought out a nurse with a wheelchair to get me into the E.R. After getting me into the wheelchair the girl who was pushing me I could tell was not that experienced. There was a paved ramp that led up to the automatic doors from the parking lot. Now I'm a big guy. I'm 6 foot 3 inches tall so in order to accommodate my height the wheelchair has an extension bar for the legs that are adjustable according to height, or in this case, length. The nurse placed my legs and feet into the proper position to push me up the ramp. Everyone outside and inside the Emergency room was about to find out just how much pain I was in. While she pushed me up the ramp, she went a bit too fast and because my left leg was fully outreached, she did not allow for the length and my foot hit the pavement of the ramp. AHHHHH!! She apologized about 10 times while still pushing me, still, a bit too quickly for the automatic doors to open fast enough. Bam! My left foot hit the door. AHHHHHH! AGAIN!! Everyone in a 2-block radius heard that one. It gets worse.

I was immediately brought to the x-ray room and many scans were taken. When they brought me back to the E.R. room they explained the damage, from what they could tell. The left leg received the brunt of the damage. My patellar tendon ruptured completely, which is why I could not move my leg. The tendon basically snapped off and rolled up like a window shade, as one of the surgeons explained. Also, the metatarsals snapped like twigs. The way it was explained to me was imagine interlocking your fingers as you join hands and then raise your fingers up. That was basically how they snapped with a few of the bones pierced through the top of my foot. Another consequence of the wall was a Lisfranc dislocation fracture. The Lisfranc is the bone that stems from the top of the foot to the big toe. Even though I lost my big toe in 2017 the bone in my foot remained. This bone fractured and popped out of the socket and was dislocated from its normal position. Oh yeah, I almost forgot That I fractured my right foot in 2 places. The least of my worries.

In order to stabilize the left leg, they had to cast it to protect it from further damage. I needed a Trauma Specialist to handle the surgeries that were forthcoming and the hospital I went to did not have one. Cringe moment on the way. In order to cast me, they had to pop the Lisfranc bone back into the socket and to make sure the snapped metatarsals were not protruding through the skin. So, the on-call surgeon put it to me simply, "We can numb your foot, but we can't numb bones. This is gonna hurt". They must have shot me with lidocaine about 20 times. He brought a surgical intern into the room to help with the procedure. They used a portable x-ray machine and they put on led garments and gloves and they held my leg still and with the aid of the machine, pushed and pulled on the bone to try to get it back into the socket. AHHHHHH! "Bite down on this towel", the surgeon said. Just like a western movie where they give a gunshot victim a piece of leather to bite down on as they remove a bullet. Only in the movies they just take out the bullet. One time. The first attempt to set the bone failed. So did the second attempt. They thought they had it on the third attempt but…..nope. Fourth time is a charm. AHHHHHH! That was unbelievably painful. They pumped me full of whatever pain killers they were using, and I was finally doped up enough to relax. The following pictures will help you to grasp the situation.

/ preface / 17

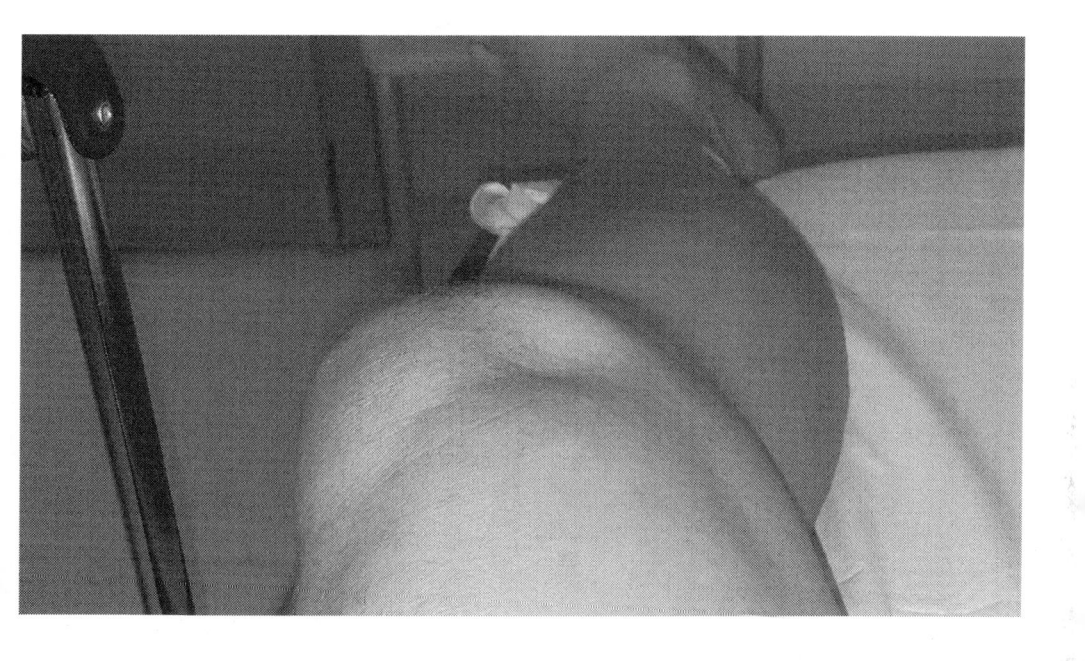

/ preface / 18

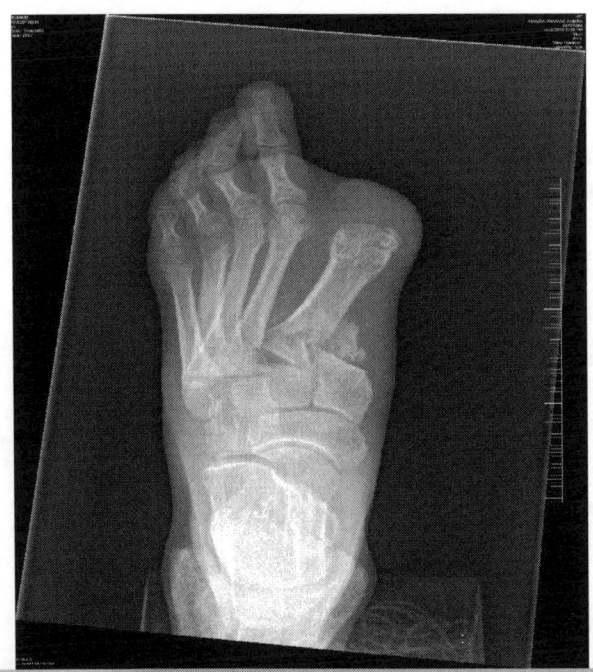

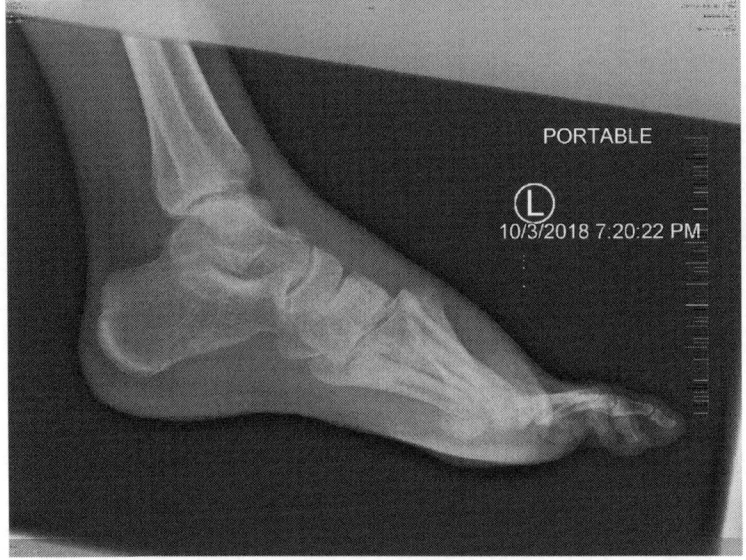

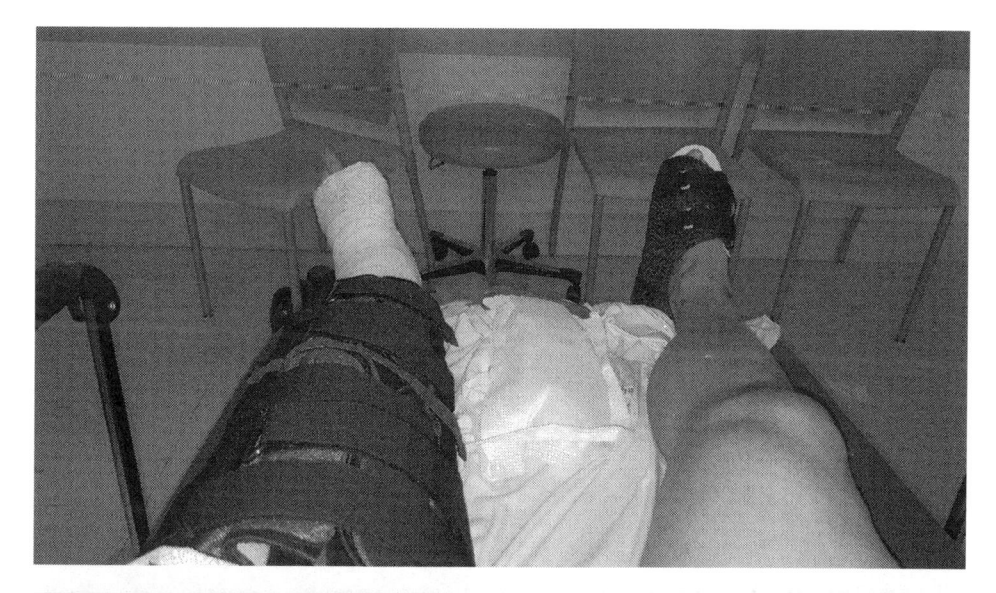

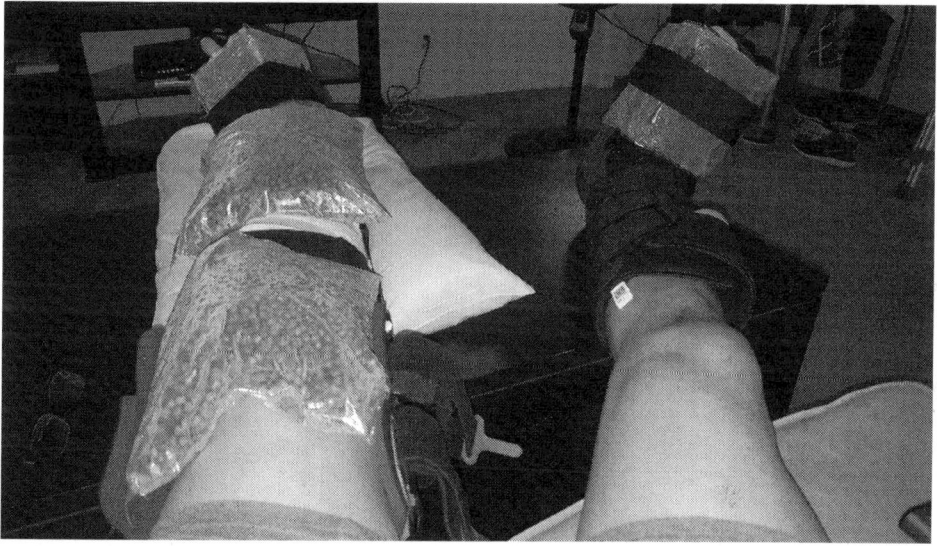

The next step was to see a specialist who could deal with this mess. With the help of my ex-girlfriend, Susan, we found a Fracture Trauma Surgeon at Penn Medicine in Philadelphia, who was an expert in dealing with such traumatic damage. Susan helped me get back to my

/ preface / 20

apartment where she loaded up my freezer with frozen peas and the ice down began. It was imperative to keep the swelling down until surgery. A few days later we went to Penn Medicine and met with the Surgeon. My cast was removed so they could inspect and do more x-rays.

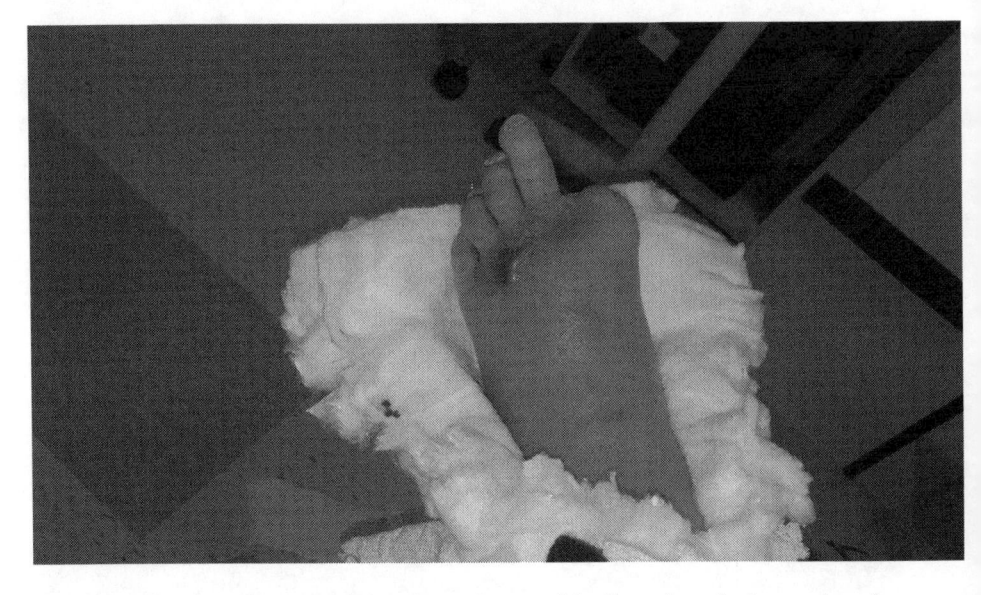

If you look closely, you can see the marks on the top of the foot where the bones pierced the skin. The welt up by the toes is a fracture blister from the breaks.

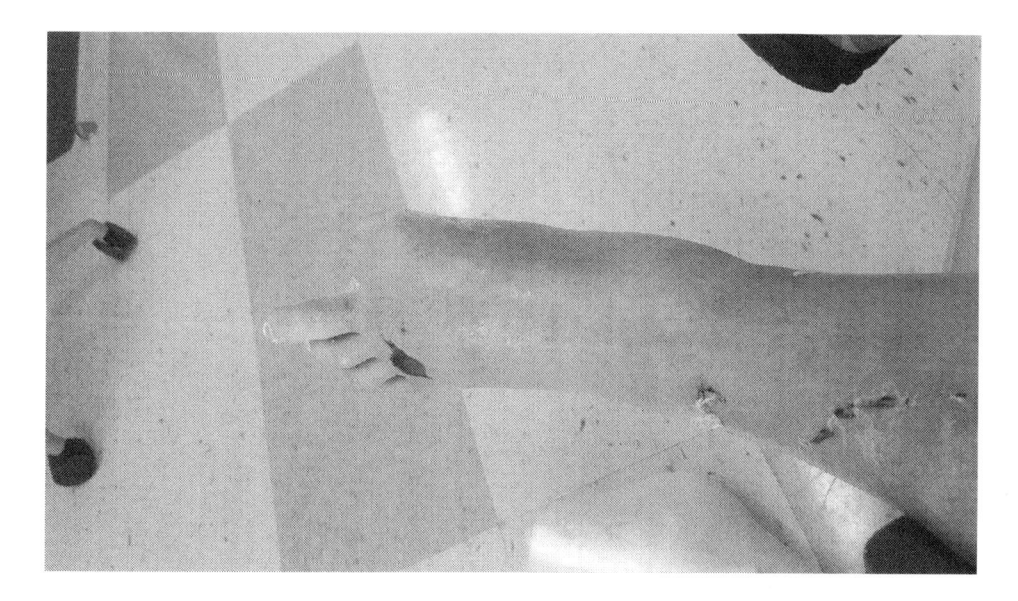

The accident occurred on October 3rd. Surgery was scheduled for October 22nd. My sister Jeanne and her husband Jim drove in from Massachusetts to go with me to the surgery and help me get situated afterwards. I was given what they call a "nerve block" to numb the entire left leg from the top of the hip down. Then they knocked me out. When I came out of surgery after 6 and a half hours, I was brought to recovery where Jeanne and Jim were waiting. Unfortunately, when I came to, the nerve block did not take, and I was writhing in pain. They did another nerve block and it finally took. The hospital kept me overnight and I was released the following day. We went back to my apartment and got my bedroom set up so I would not need to get up for anything but to go to the bathroom. The first night was brutal. Jim said he had never heard anyone in so much pain in his life. The worst of it was the nerves in my knee started to fire off and my leg was twitching. I could not control it and the pain was unbelievable. We were on the phone for a few hours with the hospital and finally got a script for Tramadol, a muscle relaxant. Took an entire day for the drug to work and I was able to rest, somewhat. Jeanne and Jim left a

/ preface / 22

few days later and I received home treatment from the hospital. I still did not know what they actually did, and I was told when I get my stitches removed it would all be explained. A few weeks later the cast cam off and stitches removed.

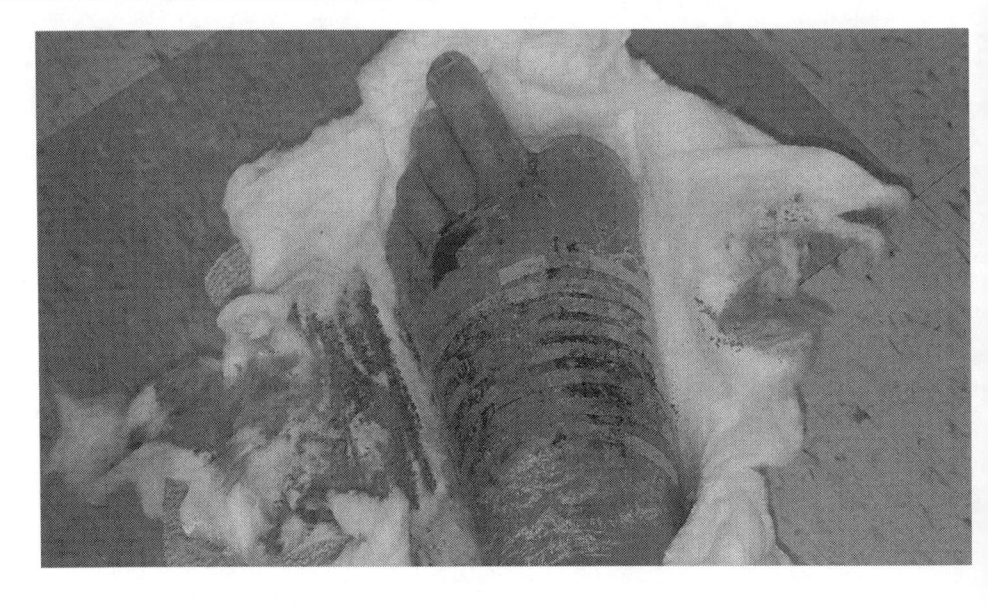

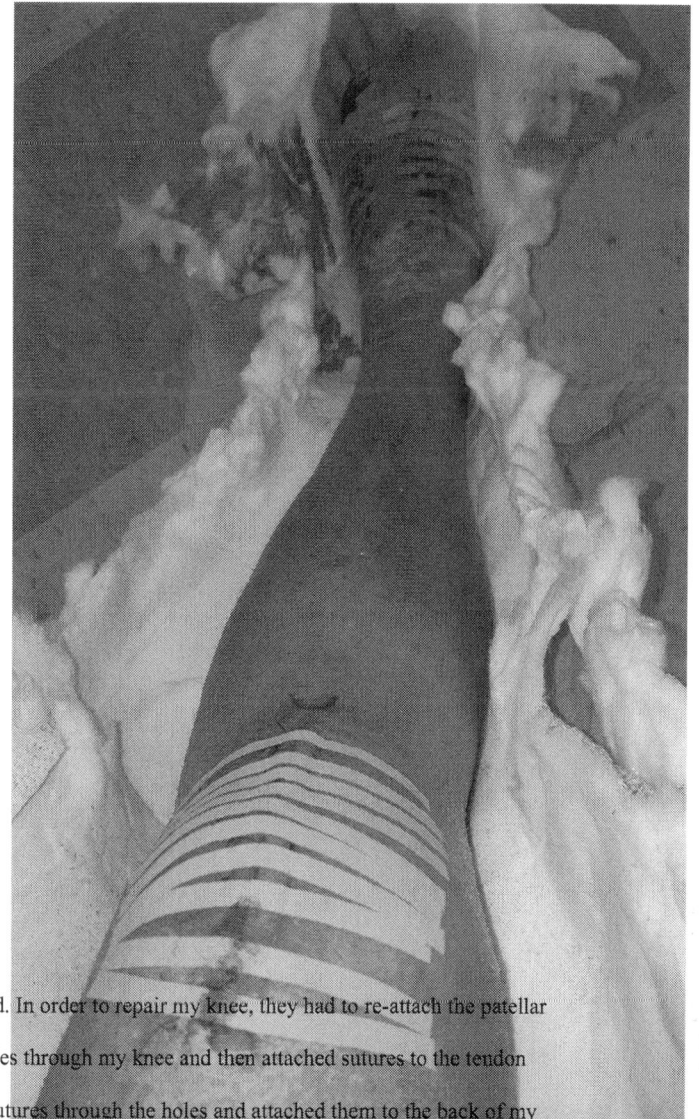

Here's what the surgeons did. In order to repair my knee, they had to re-attach the patellar tendon to the knee. They drilled holes through my knee and then attached sutures to the tendon and pulled it taut and then put the sutures through the holes and attached them to the back of my knee. The concern was to get the tendon taut enough so there would be resistance. If too loose, I would have major issues trying to walk at all. For the foot, they aligned all the metatarsals and Lisfranc within their proper position and then inserted 3 metal plates and 14 titanium screws to secure it all.

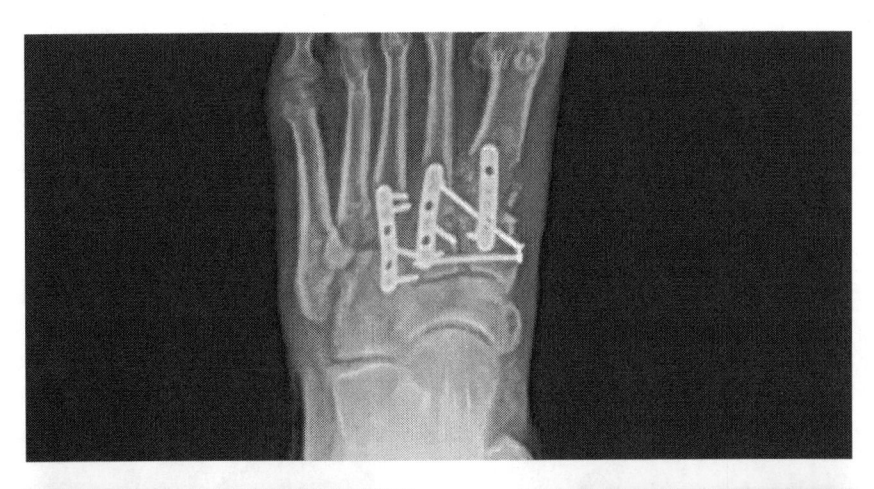

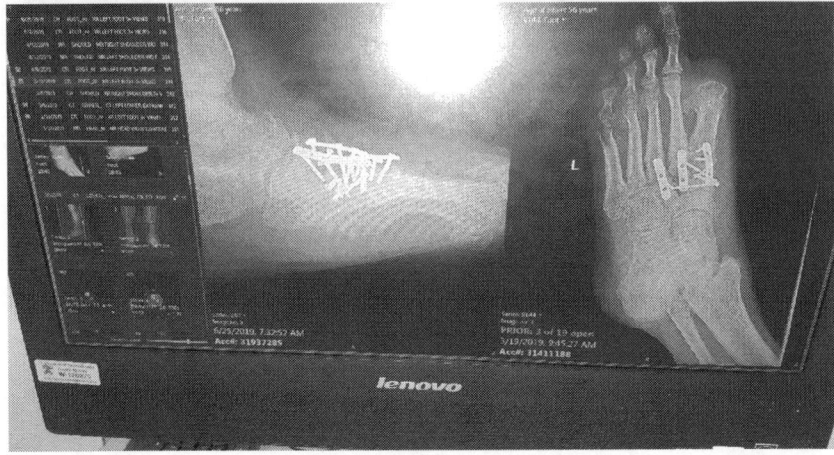

The above photo was an x-ray taken in June of 2019, 8 months after the surgery.

That x-ray from June 2019 was very significant, which I will elaborate on in a bit.

During the entire healing process, I had x-rays taken every 2 weeks to monitor how the bones were healing and to look for any issues. There were 2 incisions on the top of the foot and one long incision along the left knee. Because of all the swelling from the surgery and the fact that my foot was now "fatter" with all the hardware installed, a few of the stitches had failed and the wounds were not closing and healing. Another surgery was required to close the wounds. The next series of photos show the wounds before and after the second surgery.

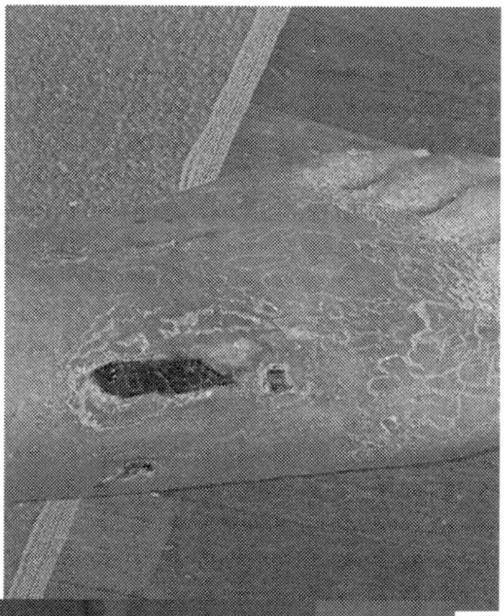

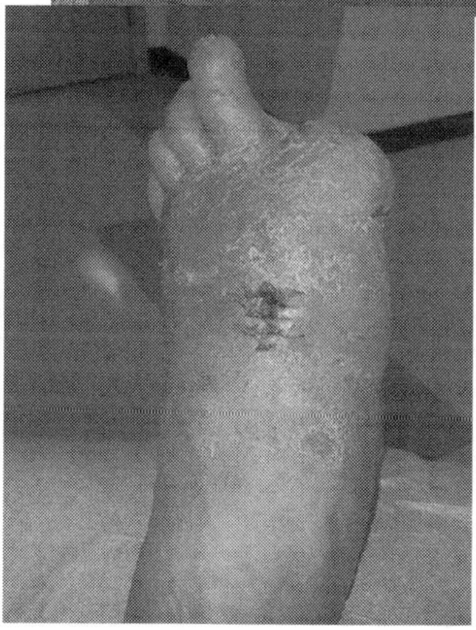

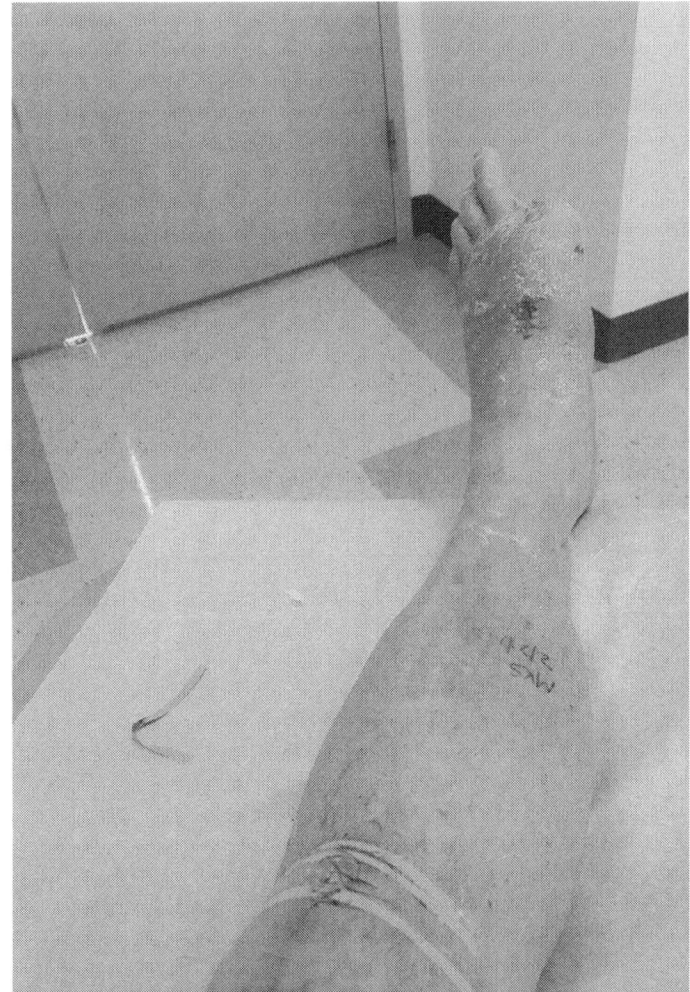

I was told at the beginning of this process that it would take between 9 months to a year for me to heal from these surgeries. I was also told that the hardware could stay in my foot for many years. But after the incisions healed my foot was always swollen. The only thing that helped was lying down. I tried to go back to work in May and June of 2019. I would pick up and drop off supplies and materials to one of my workers and I would check up on him during the day. Luckily, the jobs were close to home. After I would pop in on a job to check the progress I had to go home and lie down because of the swelling. The hardware in my foot was becoming an issue.

Now we are getting to the crux of this story. Charcot foot. I went back to my surgeon's office in July and told them I was having major issues with pain and swelling in my foot and that the pain was spreading to the bottom of my foot. After taking an x-ray the image was brought into the exam room and the surgeons PA reviewed it. I looked at the image and noted the bottom of my foot. It was kind of flat bottomed. I asked what that was all about and she said "Oh, that's the Charcot". She acted as if it was no surprise to her. It was to me. "What is Charcot"? It was explained to me that sometimes people with neuropathy and/or people who have had trauma to their foot or ankle that takes a long time to heal, can get this condition. She told me that the arch in my foot was collapsing. It was collapsing to the point where the arch was pronounced or dropped below the level of the heel and toe pad. These pictures show my arch before the surgeries and after.

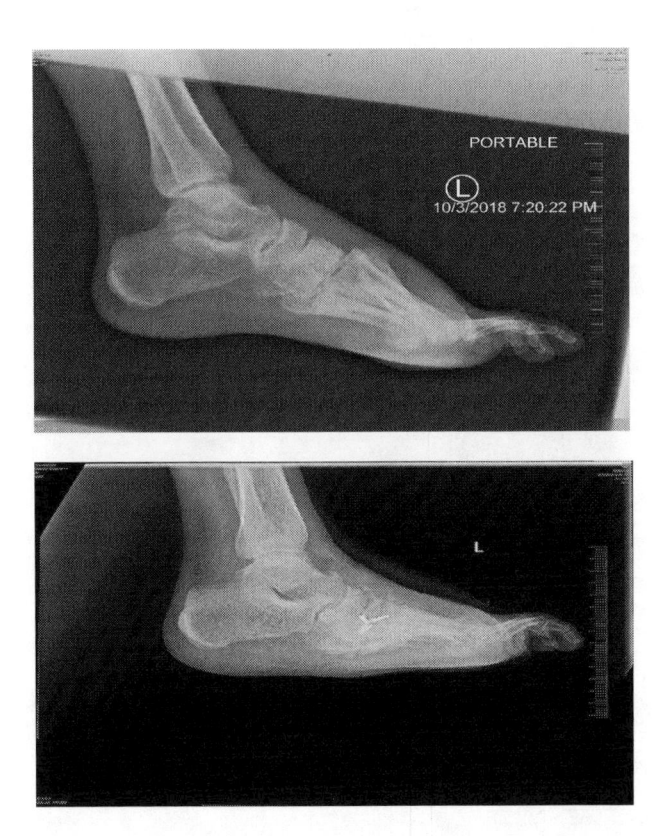

No arch. Gone. It was determined that some of the screws in my foot were backing out as well and that the bones had healed enough to remove the hardware. I had to deal with another surgery to remove hardware that they told me would be in my foot for years. Here's a picture that shows the lump on the side of my foot caused by the longest screw backing out.

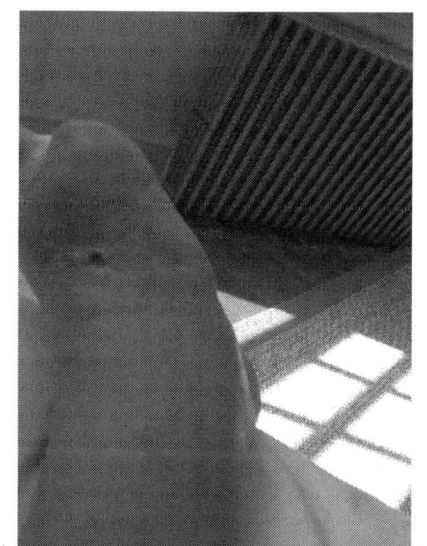

The 3rd surgery was done in August of 2019. The plates and 10 screws were removed. 4 of the screws could not be removed because they had infused into the bone. The only way to remove them would be to go in and unscrew them from the bone and then insert pins and more screws that would go though my foot from the outside and I would have to wear a brace with the pins for a year and then they could be removed. No thanks. So on with my life I went. Had to go to work because I was destitute. My brother started a Go Fund Me page and many of my friends and family donated to my cause and I was extremely humbled and thankful for all the help I received. It saved me just enough to get back on my feet. Now I just had to deal with the Charcot.

Chapter 5: 2020 Bye Bye Leg

After the drama that took place between 2018-2019, I was left to deal with the aftermath of multiple operations, most notably, Charcot foot. There were other issues that needed to be addressed such as 2 torn rotator cuffs, carpal tunnel in my left hand and a torn meniscus of my right knee. I had to prioritize so the foot took precedent. We discussed options that were available to deal with Charcot. There were 3 options available to me in making my decision, so I had to weigh the pros and cons to each option. Keeping in mind that each option would affect my quality of life. There was a lot to consider. I am a paint and home repairs contractor, and my goal was to go back to work. I met with an Orthopedic Podiatrist who explained my choices. The first step was to get fitted for an orthotic insert and shoe to accommodate my collapsed arch or rocker bottom foot. The 2nd option was to get fitted for an AFO brace (Ankle Foot Orthosis) and the final option …amputation. I agreed with my doctor that the best way to proceed would be to do the simplest thing first and see how it goes. No need to go to the extreme yet.

We went to the Foot Solutions Store and I got fitted for work boots with orthotic inserts that I could remove and place in different shoes. The problem with buying shoes at this point was that my left foot was now much wider and fatter than my right foot. My right foot was 4E width. My left foot was a 9E. Luckily, there is a website, The Healthy Feet Store, that allows you to order different sized shoes and even gives a discount for multiple purchases and has a great and easy return process if needed. The pair we ordered from Foot Solutions were a goof fit but a bit bulky of course. They served me well for a time, but the pain never went away. Keep in mind that my arch was now dipping down below the level of my heel and toes, so I was basically walking on the bones, as the recent photos show. The photos also show how swollen the skin was and here is an example of the difference in my feet sizes.

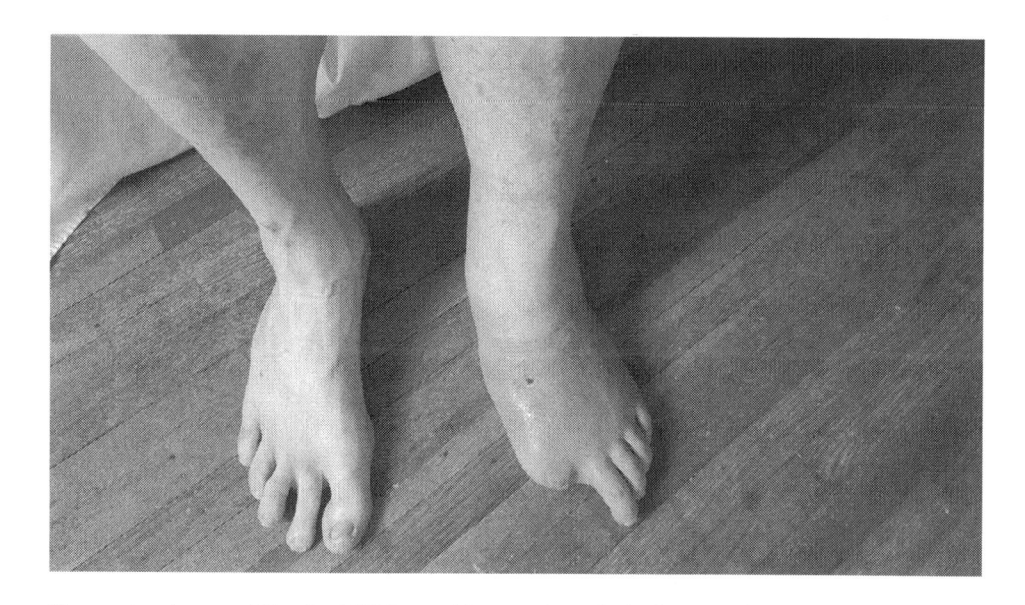

The next option would be the AFO brace. The way it works is there would be an initial fitting for this brace which basically is a plastic and/or carbon support that gets fitted to your calf and goes down the back of the leg and ankle and turns in under your foot. This brace then allows you to put on a shoe and the sole of the brace goes inside the shoe and then straps around your calf so it can absorb your body weight and thus relieving weight and pressure on the foot. I did not choose this option because the bottom of my foot would still be resting on the plastic sole, and it would not allow me to be on my feet all day. It would limit my range of motion and my ability to be more agile. I asked my doctor if I could climb Mount Everest with this brace and he said "No". "What if I had a prosthetic leg?" I asked. He said, "Yes, I think so". I was leaning towards option 3 at that point. There was another option available, but it was a non-starter for me. There is a procedure where surgeons would remove a 2-inch section of my foot and then reattach the 2 remaining sections together in a manner that would give me an arch. The healing time and recovery from that procedure would be too long and painful to endure. As luck would have it, I actually met a person in the Foot Solutions store that had this procedure done. He was in his late 60's and was an attorney. He said he had no history of diabetes but did have peripheral neuropathy that led to his Charcot foot. He said if he had the chance to do it over again, he would have not done the surgery. He said he would fall flat on his face often because his left foot was 2 inches shorter that his right foot. I'm very fortunate to have met him at that time.

In the first 3 months of 2020 I was back to work, and it was a struggle. There were a lot of external pressures on me to get back to work and pay bills. My foot was a problem. I was basically living just to work and then I could do no more. Could not go out after work and I did not go out much on the weekends because I had to spend most of my time with my foot raised to relieve the pain and swelling. Not much fun. Then, the pandemic of Covid-19 hit. And that was the beginning of the end. All work stopped for me. Jobs that I had booked for months out were cancelled. People were doing their own painting and home repairs because everybody was at home, and no one had extra money to spend on a contractor. When Congress passed the CARES Act it allowed for self-employed people to collect unemployment where they were otherwise not qualified. It saved my life because when I had the accident, I had to get out of my apartment lease because all funds dried up and I could not work. I was taken in by a friend but that had its limits and as covid hit I was asked to leave. Luckily, I had some friends who were staying at their cabin in the Poconos during the pandemic and they allowed me to stay at their place. They really bailed me out and I will be forever grateful. The work drought continued for months. I had a decision to make. The only reason I remained in the Philadelphia area was because of a relationship I was in, and I had my business there. The relationship had already ended and now that the pandemic was raging, so did my business. I made the decision that it was finally time to move back to Massachusetts and be closer to friends and family. I had to keep in my mind the fact that I would also need some support if I was going to be making tough medical choices. I packed up everything, including all my company tools and supplies, rented a truck and moved back home. My brother was also looking for a new place to live so we went in on an apartment 50/50.

Now during this time frame from the spring of 2020 to the summer of 2020, something happened to me that has never happened before. I developed and ulcer on the bottom of my left foot. I am a diabetic and I have never had any type of ulcer before as my disease has always been fairly regulated. The ulcer was a direct result of the Charcot foot. I cared for it by washing it twice a day and changing bandages 2 times a day. I spent $90 per week on bandages. Another cringe moment.

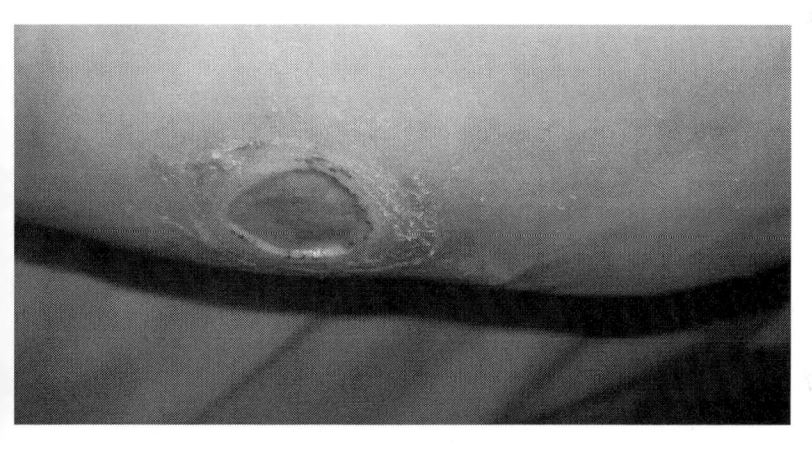

The ulcer was under control but then I developed an infection around the toe pad.

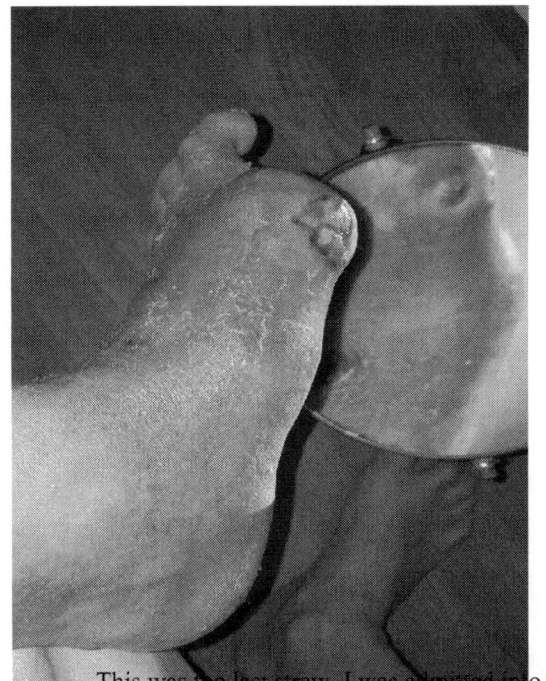

This was the last straw. I was admitted into the hospital to deal with the infection. They brought in a Vascular Surgeon to discuss my situation. I had mentally been preparing for this since the time that the hardware was removed from my foot and I developed Charcot. I tried the orthotics. I tried the special shoes and now I developed and ulcer because I was walking on a fallen arch. The surgeon told me that Charcot can stop just as quickly as it started, and it can also start up again at any time in the future without warning. If you think that once the arch collapses it can't go any further, you would be wrong. I was told the bones can easily just keep falling and ultimately go right through the bottom of my foot and even deform my ankle in the process. I've seen pictures of such deformities and they are not pretty. Another alarming side effect would be the bone shards I could possibly have to deal with. Because Charcot is a degenerative condition, the bones in my foot would become more brittle and prone to easy fractures. Because I had neuropathy and had numbness in my feet, I was told I could break my foot just walking to the bathroom, not even know it and continue to walk on it and have the bones splinter and the shards would poke the flesh inside my foot and infections would follow.

       I had to ask myself if I could deal with this every day of my life. I would now be prone to ulcers and infections for the rest of my life, let alone the intense pain that came with it. And how am I supposed to go to work every day if I can barely walk? What would my quality of life be like? The answer? There would be no quality of life at all. There would be nothing but pain and misery. I was having very dark and scary thoughts. Constant pain can do that to a person. I often thought of ending it all. Why go on? For what? Just to work to pay bills? No Life. No Fun. So many bills. IRS debt stemming from the closing business and no income. Bleak at best. I was brought to the realization that the day I had that accident, my leg was doomed. I would have done better if they just hacked it off right then and there. The toe amputation, the fall, the surgeries, the infections. One injury after another on the same leg. It was time for the dead weight to be removed. The leg was holding me back from having somewhat of a normal, pain free life. I decided to take the leap and have it removed. The surgeon was unbelievably informative in presenting a case for and against the amputation. We discussed every aspect of it. I had been doing research on my own for almost a year when considering this option. He gave me a week to think about it one more time, but I did not need to wait any longer. I had him book the surgery for a BKA (below the knee amputation).

       It's important to remind everyone that I am a type II diabetic. 1 year before my toe was amputated my A1C was 6.4. People don't realize what pain, stress and lack of sleep can do to someone's glucose levels. Throughout all my injuries during the period this book covers, my glucose levels were high. Too high. I had levels between 350-400 every day. My A1C jumped between 11-12. When I had the accident, they almost did not allow me into surgery because my blood was above 350. I had to get my doctor to sign off on it. That was a concern when I went for the BKA. My blood was 358. Even though I have had higher than normal glucose levels, I have always been a fast healer. I had the operation at the end of October 2020. The surgery took a couple of hours, and I was brought to my hospital room to recover. I had very little pain. In fact, during my initial first few days I was given a morphine drip I.V. that had an electric pump attached that allowed me to control my dosage of the drug by depressing a button that was on my bed. It was set up so that I could not overdose and allow more doses than was allowed per hour. The prescription was for 6 bags of the morphine drip, but I only went through about a bag and a half. My blood sugar taken right after the surgery dropped to 150. The pain was gone. I cried. I could not stop the tears. I was so happy at that moment to not have pain anymore. You have no idea what I felt day after day after day. Pain. Always pain. Now it was gone. That night I had to use the bathroom that was in my room. I got myself up and unplugged the monitor and I.V. and got ahold of the walker in my room and hopped to the bathroom with the monitors in tow. It was 2am. The nurse came in to check on me and when she saw the bed empty, she freaked out. She knocked on the bathroom door and asked me what I was doing. I told her I had to go. She said, "You can't get out of bed and go to the bathroom alone"! "Sure, I can" I said. "Not anymore"! she stated. And from that point on I was on the bed alarm. I tried to get off the bed a few times but was "nailed". That thing was loud.

It's important to clarify my situation as unique. Unique in the fact that I **wanted** this amputation. I wanted the pain to go away. The surgeon said that most people who get bka amputations are older people that have the procedure as a result of poor diabetes control and from sores and ulcers that get infected and bedridden subjects. I was younger and stronger than the average amputee, so my scenario was a bit different than most. After 6 days in the hospital, I was transferred to a rehab facility for physical and therapy.

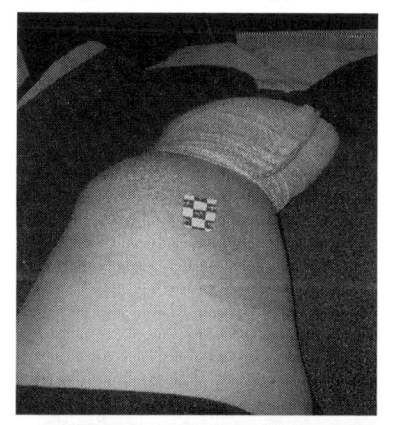

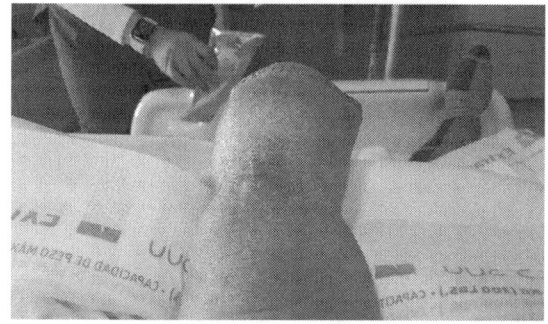

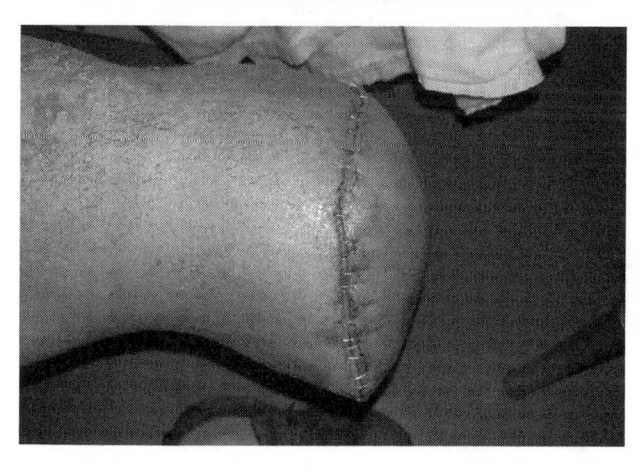

The healing process was long. After a few weeks I was allowed to go back to my apartment to recuperate. The first night I was home, I was using crutches and I went to pick something up from the coffee table and my crutches slipped off to the side on the slippery floor and I dropped straight down on my residual stump. Another cringe moment. I was doing pretty good with pain up until that point. Just Tylenol. But that hurt like hell and was another level of pain. I ended up popping a few staples and eventually had to go in for a cleaning of the wound. Since I had been taking care of my own wounds for so long, I was given instructions on how to manage this new wou

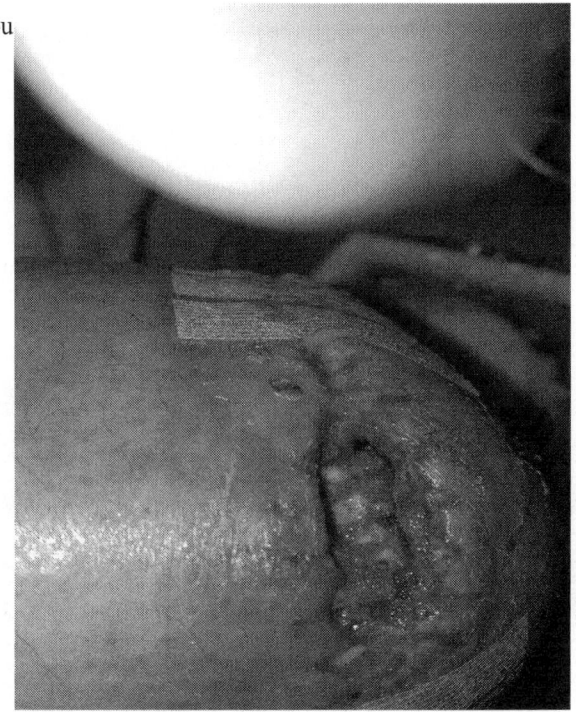

/ preface / 39

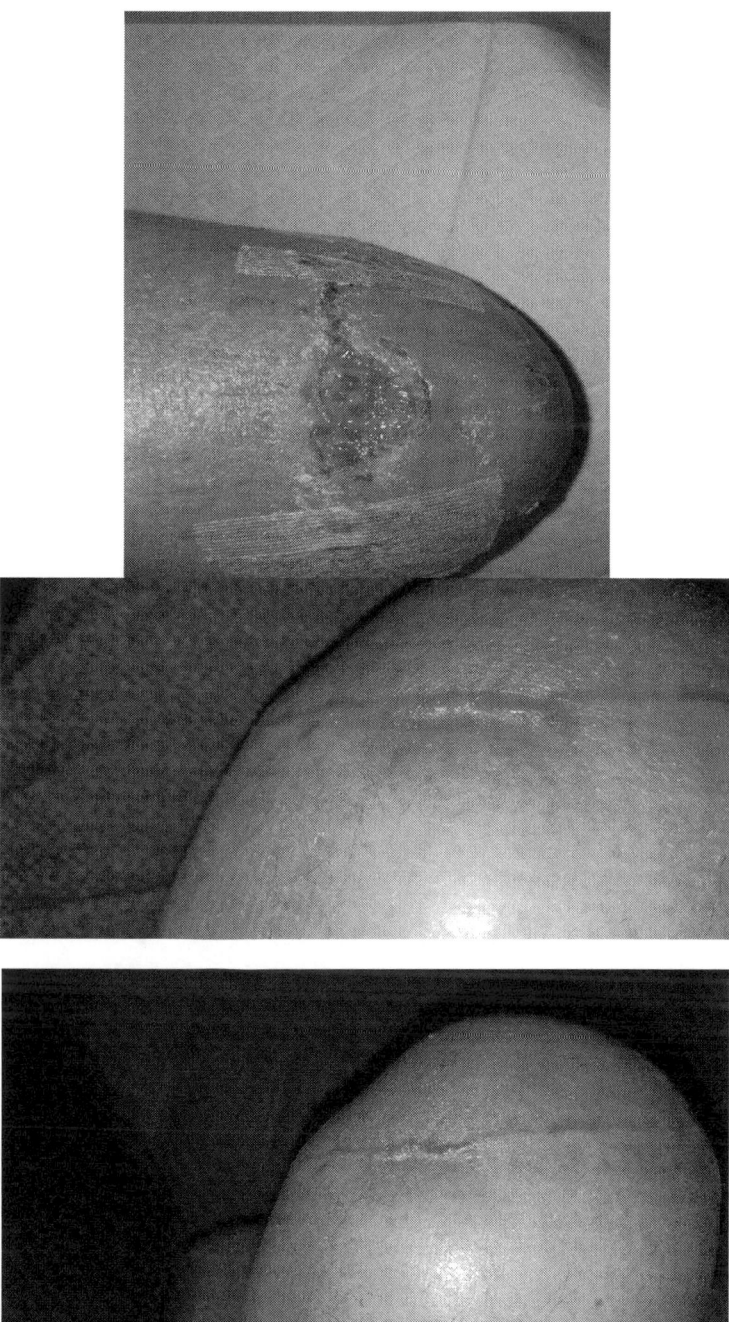

Chapter 6: 2021-present

The next step was to get fitted for a prosthetic leg. The processed entailed meeting with a specialist in prosthetic devices for consultation and a plan to prep the leg for the fitting. I was given special socks called "shrinkers" that I would put over my residual that would shrink the size of my "stump". After several weeks of shrinking the residual, I was fitted with a prosthetic that worked with a neoprene sleeve with a "pin" at the bottom that locked into the carbon shell that my residual fit in. I would wear this leg and walk on it, with the aid of crutches, to prep me for my next leg which would be the prosthetic that I have on now. It takes a lot of time and effort to get to the point of walking with no assistance. There is always pain involved but nothing like I went through before. There are still issues when I walk. My left knee is still stiff from the operation back in 2018. Stairs are a bit of an issue at times, but it gets better every day. I will always need crutches at my bedside for going to the bathroom at night when my prosthetic is off. I have a portable bench seat in the shower as I cannot get the prosthetic wet. I could cover it with a plastic leg protector but by the time I get the stupid thing on, I could just take a shower without the leg. The prosthetic weighs more than my own lower leg so you need about 20% more exertion of energy to move it. But the use of crutches over a long period of time doesn't help my shoulder situations. As I write this page today, I am recovering from Rotator Cuff surgery on my right shoulder. I have 3 surgeries remaining. The left Rotator Cuff, left hand carpal tunnel and a torn meniscus of my right knee. I take it one day at a time and will try to wrap up the remaining surgeries by early next year.

When I had the leg removed, I applied for Social Security disability benefits. I was originally denied because, according to Social Security, the loss of 1 limb does not qualify for benefits. If you lose 2 limbs, you automatically qualify for benefits. I reapplied with the help of a Social Security representative in the Boston office. He was a great help, and I really appreciated his guidance. It took 11 months to get approved. 11 nerve wracking, anxious, sleep deprived months. The benefits don't pay for much, but it helps. The best way to get out of a hole is to dig yourself out. I am striving to get back to work. I can't survive for much longer on these benefits, so I am aiming towards getting back into work shape. Can't wait. I hate being idle. That's one of the reasons I wrote this e-book.

Chapter 7: Thank You

When my brother started a Go Fund Me page, after my accident, I never dreamed that so many people would reach out to help me. Family, friends and even friends of members of my family, people whom I have never met, donated to my cause. It was and still is, extremely humbling. I am truly grateful to everyone who donated, sent me a card or a letter or an email with words of encouragement and hope. There are a few reasons why I wrote this short book. Most importantly was to inform people of the harsh realities of Charcot foot. I have scoured the internet on the subject and realized that there were not really many stories from everyday people who have this affliction. I want to let people know what their options are for treatment and what to expect as they cope with Charcot day to day. If I help 1 person, then it's worth it. I will even list an email address I set up for people to reach out and ask questions, if they have any, or for any advice I can give. Another reason for telling this story was to let people know what I went through. That there was a legitimate reason for starting a Go Fund Me page to help me out. I don't usually ask for help. I still have a hard time dealing with my feelings over asking for help. But I want people to know that what they did for me mattered. It gave me a lift when I was down and I will never forget it.

Before I had my leg removed, some people thought I should set up another Go Fund Me page, but I was against the idea. People already helped me. I did not want to whine about my situation and ask for help anymore. Times have been tough for everybody these days. It's going to take several years for me to get out of the hole, but I can do it. I just need to get back to work. Writing this book is one way to get back to work without all the physical abuse my body goes through. I will do it as a side gig unless it becomes more fruitful. Keep checking my Facebook page for updates and blogs.

There are a few down sides to getting an amputation. Some amputations are elective. Some are absolutely necessary. Some are sudden and tragic. I think about all the Veterans and the horrors they went through that ended with amputations from senseless violence and wars. Or the children that are born with afflictions and conditions that render some limbs useless and burdensome resulting in amputations. The emotions and feelings that amputees go through are ranging from depression with the reality of "what am I going to do now?" to the anxiety of "how will I do this?" and "who will help me?". I want to let them know that there is hope. There are people who will rally by your side. There are people and services out there to help people when tragedy strikes. There are countless videos and stories on line of peoples experiences with their amputations. Attitude is key. I know it's a cliché. You can get sick and tired of people saying the same thing over and over. "Keep your chin up!". "You can do this!". "Remember there are people out there that have it worse than you". Yeah. Gee thanks. That really cheered me up..lol. It's ok to feel bad. It's ok to cry. It's ok to be in a sullen mood. Hell, you've earned that right! The only advice that I can give is to just keep trying. Do not give up. Try to get out there and breathe the fresh air. Exercise, if you can. Eat the right foods. If you want a better life it starts with a better **you!** You can't be a better anything (writer, carpenter, shelf stocker, account manager etc..) until you are the best **You** that **You** can be.

Attitude is huge. I am one of a very few who absolutely had to have this surgery and welcomed it. My attitude is super positive. I **know** I can do whatever it takes to thrive. I **will** succeed. Every year for Christmas, I would send out Holiday cards for all of my clients that I serviced and my friends and family. For obvious reasons, I have not sent any over the past couple of years. This year I decided to send out just a few. I wanted to make my own cards. So, I had a card made up.

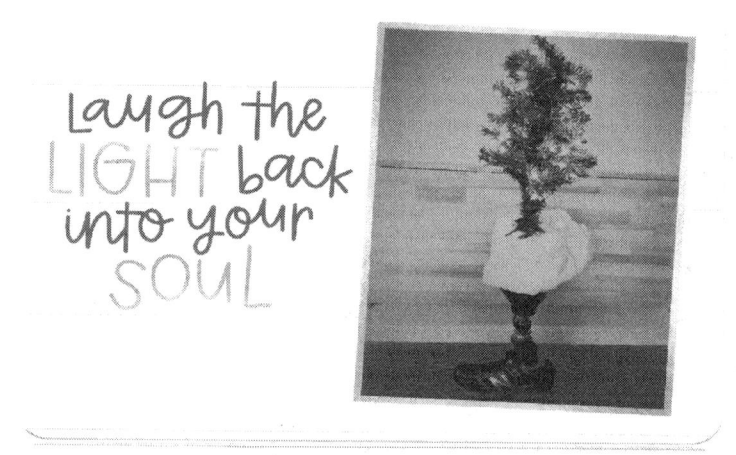

Laugh the LIGHT back into your SOUL

Wishing you all the happiest Holiday Season and a leg up in the New Year!

My prosthetic leg with a lit-up Christmas tree in it. Why not? I did it to let people know that I am ok with my situation. That the future looks bright. And not to feel bad for me but to feel joy and happiness. We all need to laugh more. Especially when things are bad, and times are tough. I want everyone to know that you will see me more when I am a better me. I still feel a bit anxious to see people I know. I want them to see me when I am standing straight and tall. When I can walk a little better and get into better shape after all these procedures. I will get there. It will take a bit more time, but I will get there.

I want to recognize a few people for their generosity and assistance during this awful and painful time in my life. When I had the accident in 2018, I was living in an apartment in Elkins Park, Pennsylvania. Just outside Philadelphia. I moved in in 2016 when my relationship with my girlfriend ended. We had been together for about 15 years, but we have known each other for over 20 years. Because my recovery was going to take over a year, my ex-girlfriend Susan, moved me into her house that was only a half a mile away. One of my workers, Gus, and my friend Mark, helped me with the move. Susan worked diligently to help me sell and remove all the furniture and items I could not take with me. The rest we put in storage where my company tools were located. She also got in touch with the apartment association and got them to release me from my lease because of my situation. Susan was the one who found the surgeon who was a specialist with traumatic fractures. We would hold a conference call with my brother Steven to coordinate and come up with a plan on how to proceed. Susan did all of this while working a demanding full-time job as she was the Executive Assistant to the CEO of a software company. She would buy all the groceries and I did all the cooking (with a walker and crutches). She helped me with several doctor appointments until I could go to them by myself. She let me take her Volkswagen to the city for appointments because my tuck would not fit in the garages in the city. My brother set up the GoFundMe page to get donations to come in so I could pay bills and survive. In early 2019 Susan was diagnosed with cancer. The doctors gave her a prognosis of treatment and an 80%-90% chance of success. I would help her by going to chemo and radiation treatments when I could but eventually, I could not go because of my leg. I felt horrible for her. 6 months after her treatment the tumor was gone, and she continued to be tested and monitored for any issues that may return. Susan saved my life. My family was 355 miles away. It was difficult for them to travel to help me, so she stepped in. Even while she was going through cancer treatments, she still had me stay at her house so I could recover and try to get back to work. I will always be grateful and appreciative of everything she did for me.

When word got out to some of my clients of my accident, they responded with kindness and generosity beyond anything I expected. That was one of the toughest things to get past. I miss my clients. They were all wonderful people, and I will miss working for them.

Now, I look to the future. I am back where I grew up and I am closer to family and friends. I look forward to spending time with everyone I missed over the past 22 years of my absence. I hope that I will recover from all issues and get back to work so I can start digging myself out of the hole I am in. My hope is that this book will be successful and leads me down a different path of work. A path that leads to more brain work and less physical work and a happy and productive life. Only time will tell.

For those with Charcot foot or anyone facing a bka or has had one and need some advice I can be contacted at; chrlyqst@yahoo.com END

/ preface / 46

Made in the USA
Columbia, SC
10 November 2024